Disclaimer

The information in this book is to assist you on your path to better health.

Although the content is based upon universal principles of health and wellness, and could provide some level of help to nearly everyone, certain individuals may have specific conditional situations that require the advice and direction of a licensed medical professional.

We advocate gradual lifestyle changes leading to permanent changes to improve health and longevity.

The content of this book is not intended to replace sound medical advice.
Consult your physician before beginning this, or any health program.

Contents:

HOLISTIC HEALTH

The
PILLARS of WELLNESS

A Mindful Path to Vibrant Health

by
Mark S. Gallagher

Also Featuring
8 Steps to Better Health
&
Inspirational Meditations

Dedication

For all who seek to improve their personal
health situation. May this work educate and
empower you to find the truths you search
for in your quest for wholeness of being and
purpose.

Introduction

Fueled by a desire to serve others of my
generation in the quest for vitality and
longevity, I began the process of developing
this book. I wanted to share what I've
learned through my extensive studies of
Chinese Qigong methods, plant based
nutrition, and the spiritual and meditative
teachings of the East. Yet for years it
seemed to lack a unifying theme.

Then one day it came - 'The Pillars of
Wellness' a simple and truthful approach to
understanding health & wellness. Three
primary arenas of health cultivated through
a balance of discipline and education,
providing insight into health patterns and
how to implement changes. Once I was able
to view health and wellness in this easy to
understand format, my personal health
began to increase and I was able to provide
a much clearer direction for friends and
fitness clients.

The 'Pillars of Wellness' is a guidebook to
the fundamentals of health and wellness in
the human body. It is a simple tool to
understand the way in, and the way out, of

many health and disease related issues. It is a complete and simple outline of what is necessary to live a full healthy life, and as a supportive text, the 'Eight Steps to Better Health' is a road map to better habits of health.

Sadly, we live in an age almost defined by poor health, in which so many diseases plaguing our culture are directly related to our modern lifestyles. Sedentary existence, poor diet and stress all contribute to individual bodily decay, as well as a broader cultural collapse of wellness values. Many of us have completely lost touch with our bodies and our health.

More than 60 % of Americans are overweight, and almost 30% obese. This has created an environment where disease has run rampant. What have we done ? In a way, we can blame the culture, but as individuals, we must rise up and take personal responsibility to implement change.

This book outlines the key components necessary to create and maintain a natural healthy state of well being. Once you begin to see health and wellness in this way, you can apply the principles to make changes in your life and begin to turn most health situations around.

It is my intention to help you reach optimal health and wellness, learn where health emerges from and take responsibility for your part in it. It all starts with opening your mind to make changes in patterns and attitudes that can provide the best outcomes regarding your health, quality of life and longevity.

Good Health starts with wanting it badly! Find your personal motivation & get going! All that matters is that you are 'on the path' and the journey has begun.
                    - Enjoy the walk !

Good Health 101

True Health is a general condition of wellbeing in body, mind, and spirit, free from disease; illness or pain, systemically in balance: the functional metabolic efficiency of a living being.

Most people have never been taught exactly what it takes to be in optimal health. They simply just trust their medical professionals to tell them what they need to do. Somewhere along the line, as western medicine grew, personal health and the basics of how to reach and maintain it, got lost in the shuffle of new technologies and expanded bureaucracies in health care.

Health Care

Too many people equate 'health' with 'health care'. Health care is for those in need of medical care, and requires a level of 'disease' or 'discomfort' to be present, requiring teams of medical professionals to assist in treatment. This process takes the personal responsibility out of the patient's hands and places it in the hands of professionals who are making 'educated guesses' based on symptoms, and seldom address the root cause.

The ethics of our health care system comes into question when you consider the elaborate profit motives of keeping individuals in chronic states of illness. The health care system is financially fed by keeping patients in a permanent disease state. If the real cures were made known, it would drastically affect the profitability of the health care industry.

Certainly, western medicine has its values, and is uncompromised when it comes to acute care. Even the pharmaceutical industry has provided us with some miracle drugs that have both extended our life expectancies and reduced the impact of certain chronic conditions.

Where western medicine falls short is in a lack of focus on prevention and the over-utilization of abrupt and chronic treatment methods. Doctors are trained in 'symptom management' and not in methods of prevention. Although some progress is being made, health care currently revolves around identifying disease, treating the symptoms and locking the patient into a systematic spiral of services, treatments, and medications for as long as possible.

If we really want better health, then we'll need to take responsibility for managing our own care. The first place to start is prevention - through living healthier lifestyles, and the second place is education - understanding the causes of illness and knowing all the options available.

What it Takes

Total health is the essence of striving to be your personal best.
Achieving total health requires a multi-dimensional approach that includes commitment, allocation of time, improving diet, finding exercise methods that can be done throughout the aging process, seeking inner peace, being focused on personal health preservation and understanding our relationships with others. All this becomes necessary to understand our whole health picture.

We each need to take responsibility for our own health portfolio. We also need to 'turn back the clock' on our dangerous health patterns. Education is the key, along with asking questions and being vigilant to seek out answers from more than just traditional sources. Individuals need to look within and assess their patterns of health to clearly reach the root cause of imbalance within their personal health situations.

Be your own health activist. Make improving your health a hobby and not a chore. Complacency will not provide you with health. You'll need to proactively 'act on' improving your personal situation. Do something good for yourself - everyday! Make it part of the 'new you', and begin to 'make choices that lead to changes'.

Understanding the basics of health and well-being is fundamental to 'tuning in' on the balance (and imbalance) within our bodies. Most of us sincerely want good health, and by following an open-minded holistic path of actively seeking the answers, we can avoid permanent 'health care', and connect to permanent health'.

Take the steps to change your life and begin on the path to a 'new you'.

Mental Health

Mental Health has to do with being in harmony with your capacity to organize life through cognitive, emotional and psychological skills. It is defined by the world health organization as:
"a state of well being in which the individual realizes his or her own abilities, can cope with the normal stresses of life, can work productively and fruitfully, and is able to make a contribution to his or her community".

The mind is developed through understanding patterns, and building that into a familiar, intuitive and innate sense. Personal development is achieved through learning pattern recognition and possibilities within patterns to an intuitive level.

An experienced person familiar with the patterns necessary to perform a defined function, attains an innate sense of cognitive skill that provides an 'intuitive edge' to easily flow through a task at hand, whereas an apprentice has yet to connect to the flow of patterns necessary to achieve full competence. This is why an experienced person, such as a nurse, is more capable of 'thinking on her feet' rather than a new graduate.

An ideal state of mental health requires the cultivation of positive resolve in both general and complex situations. A positive resolve is fundamental to all growth and depths of perception, and without it, we are stuck in a spiral of self-destructiveness.

The mechanics of positive resolve are found in the balance between conscious mindfulness and the undertones of the subconscious mind. If our 'present mind' is attempting to generate a positive thought, it requires the support of the subconscious mind to instill faith in ourselves. There are a thousand subconscious thoughts to each conscious thought; therefore the subconscious mind is a powerful tool necessary for accomplishment. We cannot achieve any level of true functional success if our subconscious mind is 'undermining' our attempts. Avoid the "I'm not good enough" and Stick to the "YES I Can !!"

Mindfulness and intention are an important part of one's mental health portfolio. They help us to keep the external world in perspective and to look within to find purpose. Finding purpose and creative expression provides us with the building blocks for happiness and a positive resolve.

When positive resolve is properly channeled it will change your life.
 A friend who recently decided to start exercising stated that, 'a daily workout can be extremely helpful to reduce depression'. How true!

Holistic Health

Holistic health can be defined as an approach to health that views the individual as an integrated system of relationships both internally and externally, rather than as separate parts. To fully understand this perspective requires looking deeply into the connections of various components within the body, mind, spirit, emotions and personal relationships.

The holistic medical method is rooted in eastern medicine, which emphasizes the connectedness of systems within the body and treats illness as imbalances within the systems. Several primary systems linked together form connected energy centers, which are responsible for regulating the flow of energies throughout the various larger systems in the body.

Disease occurs as a result of a depletion or blockage of energy flow within the body, causing system imbalances. If one system becomes depleted or blocked, the other systems drain energy to help support the weakened one. This can get complex when, over time, multiple systems become weakened and a practitioner or an individual, looks to find a 'root cause'.

Once we venture outside of the organ and cellular systems of the body and begin to investigate mind, spirit and emotion, it becomes difficult to see all the complexities within an individual.

One should always keep an eye out for the deeper connections and relationships. This requires a humble approach to always look, listen and learn.

Holistic health requires individuals take personal responsibility for their health condition. This requires making good decisions every day, and spending time learning about exactly what keeps our bodies in a 'healthy balance'.

Yes, we can work with our holistic practitioners when we are sick, and our western physicians when we need something more immediate, but ultimately we need to make our own choices and bear personal responsibility every step of the way.

About Disease

Before we address the fundamental 'pillars' necessary to achieve vitality and a healthy immune system, we need to understand the basic nature of disease. For the most part, our health picture comes down to the patterns and habits we create. When we develop 'healthy habits', good health follows. When we ignore our health or choose destructive habits, we encourage disease.

Disease is a chronic state of imbalance on multiple levels within the body.
Disease occurs when the body's natural immunities fall into extended periods of imbalance that lead to weakened states in the organ systems as well as the bio-chemical and bio-electrical systems. Over prolonged periods of imbalance and stagnation, susceptibility to disease occurs.

Many diseases can be linked to specific causes (i.e. smoking irritates lungs leading to emphysema, or diet excesses create imbalances leading to diabetes). Certain diseases seem to occur more naturally through the aging process such as arthritis,

14

circulation problems, weak bladder, etc., and some diseases simply occur randomly and seem to have no direct link to a behavioral pattern or aging process.

Disease is, in essence, a decaying situation within the body. When left alone it will continue to weaken the body. The rate of progression and severity of a diseased condition is directly related to the overall health of an individual's body and their immune system.

Prevention is the most important and first objective - well worth the time put into it.

After the opportunity for prevention has passed and an illness occurs, the objective becomes to find, address and change the patterns that may have created the root cause. When that is accomplished, the illness may be slowed down and possibly reversed.

We need to understand that certain poor lifestyle patterns can create a festering atmosphere within the body, where disease can take control and flourish.

The good news is that if we can identify the lifestyle patterns that encourage disease, with resolve and over time, we can change ourselves and our internal biochemical environment into one that encourages health and wholeness and discourages the progression of disease.

When we choose to accomplish this fundamental change, we can slow down the impact and progression of imbalances, and re-create an environment of health and wellness within the body temple. The sooner an individual can institute change, the greater the possibility for positive outcome.

We all get sick once in a while, and nobody likes to feel sick, ill or diseased.
To counter a disease progression, one must follow the holistic path outlined below.

The purpose and role of holistic health and healing is to:
1) Prevent and direct one's health patterns to avoid occurrence in the first place
2) Reverse the direction of disease and to guide it out of the body temple
3) Postpone the progression of a disease

pattern from getting worse
4) Reduce the impact a disease has on one's life and quality of life

The Pillars of Wellness

Introduction

The 'Pillars of Wellness' can serve as a guidebook to the fundamentals of health and wellness in the human body. This approach serves as a complete and simplistic tool to view overall health. It is exactly what needs to be understood in order to see the way in and the way out of health and most disease.

Almost anyone can look into the three principle arenas and see them as root causes of health and wellness. These three 'Pillars' are the primary keys to either optimal health, or sickness and disease. The choice is completely in our hands. Health and wellness comes down to the fruits of habitual patterns cultivated over extended periods of time.

The 'Pillars of Wellness' is a tool to view our current health situation, and a pathway to recovery and better health. When used as a format to institute positive change, the 'Pillars of Wellness' can be a big help in turning around a disease situation.

About 'The Pillars of Wellness'
There are three primary arenas of wellness within the body. They are interconnected and each has its own significance and place in our total health picture.

Understanding these principles is fundamental to almost all health situations. When properly maintained and cultivated, they are the **'Pillars of Wellness'** and will keep you in-health for a lifetime. When ignored through poor habits and patterns of abuse they become the **'Pillars of Disease'** and can drastically affect your quality and length of life.

The key is the immune system. The 'Pillars of Wellness' are a guide for exactly what needs to be done to your life's patterns to keep your immune system functioning at peak. All the systems in the body are important, but specifically a healthy immune system keeps us in a high state of cellular and organ system health, enabling prevention of many diseases and illness.

Each of the 'Pillars of Wellness' relies upon the others to build a balanced and healthy environment within the body. Often people mistakenly focus on only one 'Pillar', and neglect the need to keep vigilant with all three. This causes bodily disharmony. Regardless of how hard one works at an individual 'Pillar', keeping a balanced approach by focusing on all of the 'Pillars of Wellness' will yield the greatest health and wellness to a individual.

The Pillars of Wellness

1) Energy Circulation,
Keep Moving - Avoid Sedentary Lifestyle

Energy circulation is how the energy flows throughout the entire body. It includes all of our internal systems: organ systems, blood, breath, cellular, and even subtler levels such as macro and micro, bio-electrical and bio-chemical. These are all 'highways of health' in the body.

Your individual energetic signature can be crafted and developed over time. This is not something that is stuck in a 'DNA genetic formula'. YOU CAN regulate and enhance the flow of energies in your body. All it requires is a daily commitment.

Developed through Movement and Breathwork.
Movement therapies and light exercise are most effective to keep the energy flowing smoothly, and breath is the fuel for energy circulation. For those over 50, walking is great and serves as a light cardio workout. Find gentle exercise methods like Qigong,

to keep energy flowing without overworking the body. Be sure to stretch often to reach extremities. Enjoy a peaceful rest at night. Avoid the sedentary lifestyle and 'bad habits', such as sitting on the couch watching TV, smoking, drinking and excess food, which can all cause blockages to your internal energetic circulation.

2) Consumption Patterns and Nutrition,
Eat Less & Eat Healthy - Avoid Excess Weight

Modern science shows that proper consumption habits and nutrition are vitally important in the maintenance of good health, and that the Standard American Diet (SAD) is, in truth, a hindrance to good health.

You can control your weight and receive all the health benefits that come with reaching your ideal BMI (body mass index). Once you discover and believe that you can, you will succeed and overcome your self-imposed obstacles. The keys to a 'new you' are literally in your hands.

Developed through Education and Discipline.

Understanding patterns of food consumption is the first step to eliminating excess weight. Once patterns are identified, we can determine a direction and implement change. Continually making changes toward better health and weight loss is the secret. Educate yourself and learn the indisputable fact that **a nutrient dense, plant based diet is the healthiest way to eat**. Once you are 'on the path', never stop the change by reverting to old habits; keep improving your dietary patterns and you will continue to reap the benefits of good health.

By eating less volume of food and focusing on the healthiest food groups, we can put ourselves on the path to optimal health. Shedding weight is accomplished through 1) consuming less, along with 2) replacing poor food groups with healthier ones.

The highest level of nutritional health is applying the Acid/Alkaline balance into your personal diet, where the focus is on the internal chemical relations of the foods consumed. Most westerners maintain a chronic acidic imbalance that increases the body's susceptibility to many diseases.

Learn more about Acidic/Alkaline balance, and for a start: **Eat More** Fruits, Veggies, Seeds & Nuts and **Eat Less** Dairy, Meats (including fish and poultry), Processed foods, Grains and Cereals.

3) Mindfulness & Intention

Develop Positive Resolve - Reduce Stress, Depression and Compulsions

Why and how we turn our mental energies inward affects our total health and can keep us in a reflective place of peace, or bring us to self sabotaging habits that turn our willpower against us. The way we cope with our self inflicted mental obstacles such as stress, depression and compulsions can drastically affect our health, one way or the other. A positive resolve can significantly influence our situational health outcomes. The choice is ours.

We can choose to bring peacefulness into our lives by how we react to what life sends our way. The trick is not to internalize our problems and challenges. Separate and detach the original issue from the 'negative add-ons' (stress, depression, etc.) that only make things worse. When you break away from the 'self-destructive add-ons', you will have peace.

Developed through Meditation

There is nothing more effective in cultivating a positive resolve than meditative mindfulness. As a process, it **enables us to detach from and reflect upon our cognitive behavioral patterns**, freeing us from the negative impact of stress and other self-destructive mental processes (such as depression, compulsions, etc.). Mindful meditation allows us to analyze and think through our patterns of how we react, and overreact, to the world, and also develops our resolve to actually implement positive change.

The evidence is overwhelming that a positive attitude has a direct effect in achieving positive outcomes. This 'Pillar' becomes more influential as we age and develop a 'deeper knowing' that our disposition and resolve can make a difference in almost all situations. What we believe, and how we positively approach those beliefs, has a great deal to do with the way life unfolds for us.

<u>Achieving Optimal Health</u>

Optimal Health is developed through a hygiene of discipline and knowledgeable decisions, transformed into cognitive patterns of wise choices made every day.

It requires a strategy of balancing energy through the 'Pillars of Wellness' and needs to be continually developed and cultivated. If you let one aspect slide it will affect the others and their capacity to provide vitality and prevent disease within the body.

Your approach to the 'Pillars of Wellness' can span a range of internal health possibilities. There are varying degrees of health cultivation that can be attained, and each of the 'Pillars of Wellness' has a good side and a bad side. When well-cultivated and maintained, they can provide a reservoir of great health. When ignored and abused, they can turn your body into a stagnant pond, stewing disease.

Most of us fall somewhere between the poles of excellent and poor health habits. Be careful, once you begin to lean toward poor health, you may continue to fall in that direction. A lack of attention to any part of the 'Pillars of Wellness' creates potential for illness. If poor health patterns continue without positive change, simple illness can develop into disease.

Each 'Pillar of Wellness' is of paramount importance, and they are all integral parts of the whole. If we 'tune in' only to one of the Pillars and don't pay attention to the others, we are not cultivating 'total health'. Pay attention to all behavioral habits, healthy and unhealthy, as they each play a part in your internal system interaction.

The 'Pillars of Wellness' work to help each other. If you begin to lose weight, it becomes easier on your body to move and circulate energy. If you become more reflective of mind and less stressed, you will spend less time eating out of compulsion. If you stop smoking, you will breathe easier, allowing for healthy circulation in lungs and blood flow.

Throughout the aging process one must continue moving toward health improvement.

At 20 to 35yrs., one can afford to 'live a little hard', but as we age we must learn softer methods that improve overall health, and be ever more committed to a path of wellness. Vigilance and resolve will enable us to age gracefully and with good health!

In summary, reaching optimal health requires a multi-dimensional approach that includes a joyous commitment, allocation of time, improving diet, performing exercise methods that can be done throughout the aging process, seeking inner peace, being focused on personal health preservation and understanding our relationships with others. All of this is a necessary part of understanding our whole health picture.

8 Steps to Better Health

I) Commit to a better you.

II) Accept that things take time to achieve.

III) Get rid of what holds you back.

IV) Eat less & eat right.

V) Exercise & meditation

VI) Stay focused on growth.

VII) Be a spiritual person.

VIII) Preserve yourself for the long run.

It is over time and with consistency that
harmony falls into place.
The universe is patiently awaiting your wish
to regain your health.
All it takes is a firm commitment.
'Reach for the stars and they will
accommodate you'.
 Applying yourself is the only Secret!
                    - Mark S. Gallagher

I. Commit to a Better You

Take control of your path. Change your lifestyle. Make the first step now! Begin the journey by making a choice to reach for greater wholeness in your life.
YOU are the only one capable of achieving self-motivation within your existence.

As creatures of habit we fall into patterns of behavior that can entrap us. It's easy to feel we're getting nowhere and that our day-to-day existence seems to lack true fulfillment. Whether it is physical, mental or spiritual, we do basically the same things in daily and weekly patterns. When do we make time for personal growth?

By the very nature of the flow of life, all things are ever-changing. We want to cling to comfortable patterns as some kind of hedge against change, even though we know we can't escape the inevitable. We try to hide away in the mundane patterns of our lives to bypass the waves of reality that continuously bombard us with change.

Our routines and habits become our pathways. Getting through the day in that same old familiar way is easy to do. The daily patterns fall into weekly ones. Soon our whole lives are all planned out, and then out of boredom, we look for change anyway!

Choice is the Pathway to Change.
Do it now ! Make the choices that will get your health and life back on the right path. Just take the first step and begin to change a simple pattern in your life. Create positive habits: start a daily walk, join the exercise culture, become vegetarian or vegan. Make a change and move forward!

One positive change with a little self-motivation, can start a snowball effect into many more positive changes in your life. By growing through one positive change, other doors will open. Before long, you can cultivate personal growth into every aspect of your life and lifestyle.

Your health is the most important thing you have. Without it you have nothing. You can't just buy more. You can only develop it through intention, motivation and creating positive changes. You have only *now* to make the commitment to improve your situation. Every day you wait, the journey back becomes a little longer.

II. Accept that things take Time to Achieve

A commitment of time properly directed is rewarded by allowing us slow and gradual improvement. It took time to get into your current physical condition and circumstances, and it will take time to regain control of it. Make time for a better you now!

Time lets us view the effects of what we do. Many of us slowly poison ourselves by making poor choices relative to our health. These patterns often go on for years, then we wonder why we feel bad every day. If we look back to see clearly how we got here, we can understand that our life's patterns work through time to manifest us into who and what we are now.

Time is also a great healer. It can make us into who we want to be. If we focus our lives toward better health, what we seek will slowly fall into place. It requires a journey, but what fun in life would there be without 'the journey'?

You may believe that better health is somewhere in the future, and with that philosophy, you will always leave your success in the wrong place – tomorrow. You can never achieve success if you are looking only into the world of tomorrow. It is equally foolish to live in the future, as it is to live in the past.

What is required for a new you to emerge are ever increasing lifestyle changes that demand focus in the now- every day - beginning today. Choice is the Pathway to Change! Once you get control of this, things will fall into place faster than you ever imagined. Doorways will open for you to realize your aspirations.

They say timing is everything in life. Use time as a tool to accomplish what is needed on your path. Now is the time! The moment is at hand. Don't waste it. Use your time wisely and it will treat you well. Cherish every moment!

III. <u>Get rid of what holds you back</u>

Is it more than just your personal health habits? Is it your job that holds you down, or your relationships that frustrate and repress you? Does time hold you back? Then make the time to move forward! Forgive those you seek to blame. Get rid of the excuses for your lack of motivation, and find the inspiration to move on towards a better you. Go forward now!

We have developed lifestyles that saturate us with stress. Whether it comes from work, relationships, family, inside or outside, we need a tool to reduce the impact of stress on our bodies and our entire lives. By implementing change we can begin to hedge the stress in our lives.

It's difficult to acknowledge habits that hold us back. It requires deep responsibility to accept that we have developed personal habits and/or associations that are obstructing us from being where we want to be. Find harmony with your emotional self and assess the situation with a clear mind.

Be aware of destructive habits; they are the limitations most important to break free from. Put time into developing the changes you need in your life. Create positive habits that represent the person you want to be, and replace the bad habits that are holding you back. This applies to more than just personal habits; it works into relationship patterns as well.

Self sabotage is among the worst of the destructive habits we practice. We sometimes 'shoot ourselves in the foot' as we attempt to progress. Through reflection and meditative mind we can discipline ourselves to get past this odd yearning to self-destruct. Find forgiveness when you do, but hold temperance to your path and you will elevate past self destruction and move onto true cultivation.

In relationships, it can get complex to ask someone to accept your need to change, when they are usually not ready to accept change in their own lives. You need to carefully think out your objective, then execute a game plan. Take your time and be sensitive to others around you, especially family.

Don't fall prey to manipulation. There is a balance somewhere. The people who don't want you to move forward will want you to sit with them on the 'sidelines of life'. Don't waste time in debate. Commit to a better path and begin the steps to effect the choices that lead to changes. Get up and move forward!

Breaking ties is part of a 'choices make changes' philosophy that empowers you to use your valuable time in ways that are most beneficial to your health-focused objectives, which ultimately lead to a deeper harmony with our purpose.

Don't be self-centered. You must be responsible and loving on the path. Be sure that your quest is focused on self-improvement. That will create a strong link between your personal goals, family, work place, and community. When performed with proper intention, your positive changes will also lift up those around you.

If you are truly committed to a better you, then you'll need to 'take the walk' of change. Think through how much time we really have as aware beings in this world.

How do you want to spend that time? If there is a path you must be on, then take the steps necessary to get there.

Find constructive utilization of your precious moments. It all comes down to time management. How much time is wasted on bad habits? Breaking most habits is usually accomplished in three to four weeks for most people. Do something positive - you'll be happy you did. Take time for a 20 minute walk and a light healthy meal.

TRY THIS AFFIRMATION: 'The person I am makes time for light exercise, eats light and right, maintains integrity of character, treats others with compassion, and enjoys the simplest of life's pleasures' - and then acts on it!

IV. Eat Less & Eat Right

Make 'Eat Less and Eat Right' your mantra for weight loss and nutritional healing. Always refer to it and use it to shape your conscious and subconscious thoughts about your food consumption patterns. As a practical mantra, it is the most simple way to escape from the trap of poor health from excess weight.

Depending on the source, up to 65- 75% of all disease is linked to improper diet. That's diabetes, heart disease, stroke, many cancers, arthritic conditions and more. This is serious stuff. Stop playing around with what you eat! Be responsible for your habits.

Eating for Good Health.
Pillars of Wellness Number Two: 'Patterns of consumption and nutrition' are a big part of the puzzle in instituting long-term change patterns. Establishing responsible patterns in the category of diet is fundamental to implementing healthy change in one's life.

To be clear, the term 'diet' is a reference to your complete nutritional habits. Diets are what we eat, not a temporary attempt for a quick change that may deliver short term results that we often want to break out of before we even get started.

Simple as it gets, you are what you eat. If you drink milk then you absorb the energy of the cow, if you eat beef then you internalize the bull, if you eat pizza then you accept the bread and cheese to influence your internal energy. Learn from the health food people and eat light health producing foods like veggies, fruits, seeds, and light grains, and start to eliminate the foods that make your body work hard to digest such as meats, dairy, oils, salt and processed starches and sugars.

This is a hard concept for people to absorb, but the choices made regarding diet are the roots to your internal bio-organ systems. You need to know that a <u>poor diet kills</u>, or can drastically shorten life! Stop killing yourself slowly! Think of the awful patterns of poor diet repeating itself day after day, and year after year. Do people know what they're doing to themselves? They act like children getting away with something. Eating irresponsibly is foolish and will catch up with you -if it hasn't already. Please, respect your body.

Everybody knows it, but few people have the courage, sense, or understanding to make better choices that will institute healthier changes, especially regarding food consumption. I know it can be hard, but if you choose not to be on this path toward a healthier, lighter diet, then the other pillars of health can't fall into place, and you won't achieve vitality, health, and longevity.

Learn to enjoy eating and drinking less. You cannot continue to eat excessive amounts of foods that are out of balance with our humble human needs. We obliterate ourselves with fats and processed foods to excess. Consequently, on the most basic level, our cells get over loaded with garbage. Year after year, this leads to increasing susceptibility to illness and disease. What are we doing to ourselves? Have we forgotten that our bodies are temples?

By always tweaking the patterns of what you eat and how much, you will create an opened minded and disciplined behavioral pattern that will reduce your weight and bring better health into your life. Educate yourself and learn the indisputable fact that **a nutrient dense plant based diet is the healthiest way to feed ourselves.**

It comes down to a lifestyle approach requiring education and discipline. Learn all you can to make healthy food choices and develop 'keystone habits' such as daily exercise, vegetarian lifestyle, lite snacks, etc., and that will help create the will power to fuel change and slim down your weight.

Important to Note:
Feeling Tired ?   A lot of human vital energy is wasted in the digestion of foods. Ever wonder why you have no energy? It's possible that you're exerting too much energy on digestion.

Exercise & Weight Loss:
Exercising alone will not take your weight off. Regular exercise such as daily walking, will definitely improve your metabolism, which is helpful in processing the foods you eat. Exercise, although essential to good health, is only a part of the picture, and not the key ingredient for weight loss.

Example- Light exercise burns off about 100 calories for every mile walked, and 3,500 calories = one pound. So you would have to walk about 35 miles to lose one pound of fat. Start walking- or find a better way - EAT LESS !

The Weight Loss Answer:
The only way to lose weight is to reduce your caloric intake!
There are no magic pills. If you consume less you will eventually weigh less.
It's that simple. There is no other way. It is the only answer.

Calories and weight loss:
It varies slightly with body type, but if you take your weight and multiply it by 11 - that is how many daily calories you need to maintain your weight. So, if you want to weigh less, take your desired weight and multiply it by 11, and that is the calorie range you should consume on a daily average to reach that weight.

Eating less calories is the only answer to the weight loss equation. Eat more foods that are low in calories like salads, fruits and veggies. Cut back, slow down and eventually eliminate foods highest in calories and poorest in health, such as oils, sugars, fats, cereals, bread, fructose syrup, meats, dairy, chips, etc.

It takes a lot of 'not eating' to become trim. Learn to enjoy your periods of not eating as much as the time you spend eating foods. No one enjoys the bloated feeling after a heavy meal. Keep a delicate balance between your feelings and comforts regarding eating and not eating. Enjoy them both!

V. Exercise & Meditation
For Health Cultivation and Stress Reduction

"As we age, we must learn softer exercise methods that improve flexibility, joint function, balance and overall health."
Mark Gallagher

The goal of fitness and meditation is to put yourself in 'the zone'. A place of mindful awareness when consciousness dissolves into movement flow and the energies of the Body, Mind and Spirit fall into balance, creating a joyous euphoria.

Exercise
Proper exercise is a key long-term ingredient to vitality, longevity and optimal health. Exercise methods must be followed throughout life to enhance a fuller enjoyment of your time in this body. It needs to become a permanent habit and not something you do and stop when you 'lose the weight', or 'gain the strength', or 'feel good again'.

As the first 'Pillar of Wellness', energy circulation in the body is crucial. Find an exercise method that is comfortable for you through the aging process. Exercise and breathwork are a crucial path that must be done throughout your lifetime. Stay on the course.

Be careful not to commit to an exercise method that is high impact and physically stressful on your body. This might be 'OK' when you're in your twenties, or even your thirties, but when you start to go past age forty, things change. Many people think that their aging bodies can handle high impact exercise methods such as running, basketball, baseball, and karate, only to find themselves developing chronic injuries such as bad knees, ankles, back, wrists, shoulders, hips, and neck. Through repetitive and harmful patterns, your injuries will only get worse. Make exercise choices that will lead to a better feeling you.

'Soften up' your exercise methods as you age. Listen to your body's signals. There are differing viewpoints about sweating. Some suggests that too much sweating is not good for you. Heavy sweating is the body's way of reacting to excessive physical stress, an indication to slow down. Your body's way of letting you know it's reaching a stage of exhaustion and depletion. So avoid sweating too much.

You don't have to give up your current exercise routines completely. If your current exercise brings you joy without a high risk of injury, then keep at it. Also try to work a soft exercise method into your fitness practice and plan on increasing your time commitment to it as you age.

Walking is by far the best and simplest exercise anyone can do. It is low impact, aerobic, stress reducing, fun and enjoyable. Try adding mindfulness to your walking by enjoying the little things (houses, gardens, people, etc.).

Qigong offers many soft exercise methods that are low impact, relaxing, and enhancing to internal health. It also cultivates flexibility, balance, coordination, attentiveness, gracefulness, strengthens posture and improves circulation and awareness.

Meditation

Reflective meditation is necessary to find emotional balance and to accept our purpose and place in this world. It also helps us to understand ourselves and contemplate who we truly are.

The most important gift of meditative mindfulness is the development of a positive resolve. This affects health on so many levels, but specifically in the workings of the subconscious mind. It's easy to direct the conscious mind, but when we venture into the hidden world of the subconscious, we may have fear-based doubts that can throw the whole train off the tracks. Be aware of self doubt and stay focused in the positive realm. Your attitude determines your altitude!

The third 'Pillar of Wellness' is Mindfulness & Intention.
When performing a fitness method, try to work in meditative mindfulness. A meditative component will help to develop positive resolve and emotional well being, paramount in preventing stress and depression.

There are two primary approaches to meditation.

Passive or Static Meditation: The most basic and direct method is traditional sitting or standing meditation where the focus is on breath and clearing mind chatter. Learn to spend time in meditation every day. It will put your life in order, detach you from your ego and connect you to your higher self. This stuff works -don't miss out!

Active Meditation: Many fitness methods can develop mindfulness through awareness in movement. This approach requires that you 'put it into your workout', otherwise it gets overlooked. So, slow down and pay attention! Enjoy your exercise time; smell the roses, keep moving and find your peace within.

Also consider: 5 to 10 minutes for a meditative reflection after a workout.

Benefits of Mindfulness: A good exercise method should reduce your day-to-day stress and bring you to a place of peace. Stress reduction is about your body, mind and spirit. When you achieve meditative mindfulness your body will feel better and bounce back faster; your mind will reach deeper to ponder solutions, and your soul will fly higher with a greater sense of inner peace.

VI. <u>Stay Focused on Growth</u>

 As long as the mind, body and spirit are growing and focused on progress, you are moving in the right direction. Don't become stagnant. Forgive yourself if you slide back, but be ever-mindful that you are committed, and 'stay on the path' to a better you – no matter what!
With that in mind, you will have the resolve to overcome the obstacles.

When you look back on the 'best times of your life', you will most likely reflect upon a time when you were immersed in growth, maybe school days, or when you first discovered love, or learned to cultivate your professional skills. These were growth cycles that forged you into the person you are.

The 'growth cycle days' were the times in our lives that we stayed on the course and accomplished something worth the effort. These were the core cycles of working through what seemed at the time, to be a rough road ahead. Unsure how it would turn out, we knew that either success or failure was waiting at the end. In spite of the risk, we took the chance and now reflect warmly on our courage to overcome the obstacles.

When we get through growth changes, we become often better people due to the experience. Positively handling change is the way to break through cycles of awkwardness into confidence and strength. Choosing the healthy path requires breaking away from stagnation and focusing on growth. We must be motivated to find new places to grow towards.

Once you see your footprints on the path of growth, you'll discover how feeling good can be a magnificent motivator. From that point on, just 'keep on truckin.'

There is always an air of excitement at a college or a gymnasium, because of the shared feeling of growth. Each part of the whole is immersed in the pursuit of improvement. As you lift yourself up toward a better you, look at the healthy people and realize that you are becoming one of them. No amount of money can buy the feeling of accomplishment that comes when you find the motivation within

yourself (body, heart and soul) to reach toward being your personal best.
Once you get that feeling, everything else falls into place.

Embrace the growth cycles! It took a long time to slip out of shape, and it's going to take some time to get back into that place of good health. Enjoy the choices you're making today, as they will lead you to the changes of tomorrow.

VII. Be A Spiritual Person

In order for you to achieve anything in this lifetime you must be in tune with the Tao, the grand flow of all things. When you reach a point of harmony, the doors you seek will open. Of course, there are costs for such requests. This requires finding a pathway toward enlightenment, and as the old saying goes, "enlightenment doesn't care how you get there".

There are many ways to get to the same enlightened place. Regardless of what anyone tells you, there is no 'one correct path'. Be open minded. If a method works for you, feel good about it, and realize it may not work for everyone else. Draw your own conclusions: don't force your beliefs on others, and don't let others push their ways on you.

Set yourself on a course of truth and compassion, and enlightenment will emerge when you are ready. It is not something to achieve and then move on; but rather a path to be walked each and every day anew.

The first step is truthfulness. Find and know your truth within. Understand that there is flexibility within truth and everyone has their own individual truths.

Follow the loving path. Give of yourself. Find harmony with the creative energy; that is the eternal quest. Be cautious and prudent with your life's energies. Help others whenever possible. Stand strong when your heart is stirred, yet be flexible enough to adapt. Love all of God's creatures. Maintain humility, knowing that we are all part of the same 'eye' viewing the world from the 'human perspective'.

See the most gentle and loving things from varying viewpoints, and blend them with your experience of the creative force of life, and 'eureka: the kingdom of heaven is at hand!' It's that simple. Often just a state of mind is all it takes to get there. Create that peace within and around you, and pass it on!

Seek out emotional balance. Find pathways that don't step on others. Avoid getting worked up over little things. Even the big events require calm and peace of mind to reach a depth of comprehension. To reach emotional balance one must walk a path of peace and understanding.

View others with honest curiosity. Don't let them trap you into 'their side' of an issue. See things clearly and don't prejudge. Always avoid the karma of violence and suppression, and don't support those who seek to harm and destroy.

Know there is balance and gravity in the flow of life's energy. There are cosmic harmonies always flowing in and out. We shape the world around us, and we are shaped by the world around us; this is called co-creation. There is a weight to all of our actions that affects the many worlds in which we live, in one way or another.

Be a person of virtue, sincerity, and honor. Follow the pathway. It will get you there, and it will get you back. Be a beacon of light. Know that your perspectives shape not only your reality, but also shape the reality of those around you. Your viewpoint matters through your spheres of influence. Make it count for something worthy.

Know that kindness is the key to open love

in the hearts of all. It is a 'keystone habit' to achieve harmony in all your relationships. As the great Wayne Dyer says, "Ask yourself: do I want to be right, or do I want to be kind? Always choose kindness!"

VIII. <u>Preserve yourself for the long run</u>

Like a sculptor chiseling on a block of marble, your lifestyle determines your longevity. If you live too fast, you risk a fast short life. Keep your mind focused on the soft, slow pathway and life will rise up to meet you at that place.

Being on the path toward preservation is the last ingredient needed to grasp the 'golden ring' of life. When you understand how important and limited our bodies are, you will see that working the moments effectively will yield the grandest of experiences.

Youngsters often behave in self-abusive manners that burn themselves out at an early age. We have all seen the neighbor who seems so old before his time. A hard life with no desire to hold firm to true vitality often leads to a quick burn out. Don't go there! Take control and move slowly toward where you need to be.

It is paramount to develop a strategy for longevity throughout life. There are many things that can be done in a gentle manner to conserve energy. Slow down and smell the roses! Be easy on your body. If health and happiness is your goal, then it all counts in the long run.

Adapt lifestyle changes that conserve your life force.
Qigong and other yogic methods are among the most fun and easy-to-do health exercises one can learn. Find a good teacher and begin to understand how important being 'in touch' with your vital energy is to your preservation and health. Light walking also works to connect you to your health.

Preservation is about 'tuning in' to your personal health. It's not about cutting back on fun. It's about having fun and working within the natural harmonies of your life's energies. It is about knowing that hurting someone isn't going to bring peace, that one more alcohol drink isn't needed, that 70 MPH might be too fast, and that the extra slice of pizza is too much. It's knowing and feeling that when your body is being pushed too hard, you need to slow down. It's finding the place inside your heart to give and receive love.

Prevention is the pathway to preservation. By making time to improve your health NOW, you are securing a more solid base for tomorrow. The work pays off every day. Exercise routinely, eat right and work to attune yourself in every way.

Inspirational Meditations:

Unconditional Love
by Mark S. Gallagher

If we are to attain true peace, we must know that the divine flow of the life force is truly in control of our fate. Once we see this clearly, we have no choice but to trust, so why not? This very moment, put down your shield and yield to the love. Be kind to all in your path.

Love the person you are and love the people around you. Accept them for who they are. Loving yourself is a necessary ingredient for you to advance as a person in this lifetime. Find the strength within and you can change yourself into whoever you want to become. Don't stop trying, and the loving path will accept you.

Don't blame others for holding you back, when you have the power to walk your own path. Our part is to approach the world with trusting love. Even within the darkest of situations, there is a greater meaning hiding behind the obvious.

Understand, that no matter how hard you try, you will not be able to change others if they are not ready to accept change. Everyone follows their own path. Pay attention to your path and treat others with compassion as they follow theirs.

Act out of love and never out of fear. When we let fear in, it pushes love out. Don't be afraid to step forward and institute personal changes. Make sure your motives are based in sincerity and love. "Trust in the universe and it will provide".

The Power Within
by Mark S. Gallagher

"The Tao is immense, the universe is immense, the earth is immense, and man is immense". Find the power of all within you. Realize that you are part of all things, that you draw your very life's energy from all that there is. Attain oneness, accept your part with honor, humility, and kindness for all life. Cherish every moment. Carpe diem!

Know that there is great balance and gravity in the flow of life's energy. There are cosmic harmonies always flowing in and out. We shape the world around us, and we are shaped by the world around us. There is a gravitational weight to all of our actions that affects the many worlds in which we live, one way or the other.

Be a person of virtue, sincerity, and honor. Follow the pathway. It will get you there, and it will get you back. Be a beacon of light. Know that your perspectives shape not only your reality, but also the reality of those around you. Your viewpoint matters through your portals of influence. Make it count for something worthy.

Pathways
by Mark S. Gallagher

There are many paths that will lead you to the same place.
You must find your own 'special pathway' to reach your higher quest.

Follow the loving path; give of yourself; find harmony with the creative flow. This is the eternal quest. Be cautious and prudent with your life's energies. Help others whenever possible. Stand strong when your heart is stirred, yet be flexible enough to adapt. Love all of God's creatures. Maintain humility; understand we are all part of the same eye that views the world from the 'human perspective'.

Take the most gentle and loving things from varying viewpoints and blend them with your experience of the creative force of life, and eureka: the kingdom of heaven is at hand! It is often that simple. Just a state of mind is all it takes to get there. Create that peace within you and around you and pass it on!

About the Author:

Mark Gallagher is a Qigong fitness & weight loss: author, educator and enthusiast. He is the founder of Vitalitydvds.com and Sparta Tai Chi, and has owned and operated health and healthcare businesses.

Through Vitalitydvds.com, Mark produces DVD's and books on: Qigong Fitness, Zen Meditation, Weight Loss & Nutritional Healing.

Through Sparta Tai Chi, (Spartataichi.com) Mark offers: Group Classes in Qigong, 'Qigong Personal Training', Weight Loss programs, Workshops and Lectures.

Mark's 'ZEN POWER Training' workshop, has been presented at many Qigong events including: National Qigong Association (NQA) 2014 Annual Conference, and the Master Jou Memorial Festival 2014

Mark is a member of the: National Qigong Association (NQA), USA Health Preservation Association and the Tai Chi for Health Community. He is a student of Master Teachers Dr. Christopher Viggiano,

Jianye Jiang, Yuzhi Lu and Dr. Paul Lam.

Mark is a devoted practitioner of Qigong energetics including: Wild Goose Qigong, Animal Frolics, Health Preservation forms, Sun style Taiji, Baguazhang & Zhan Zhuang Meditations, and follows the 'Three D's of Qigong' practice: Diligence, Dedication & Daily.

He is a spiritually minded individual following a path of kindness and a Member of the Institute for Spiritual Development in Sparta NJ.

Mark is also a Holistic Weight Loss & Nutritional Health enthusiast.
Designing a '4 Session weight loss' program to help individuals CHANGE lifestyle habits by focusing on Health-based choices. Mark has produced two DVD's on weight loss, and offers several DVD's and books on Nutritional Healing through VitalityDVDs.com.

Friend Mark @
Mark S Gallagher on Face book